Essential Oils

Essential Oil Massage Techniques For Beginners: Prevent Headaches, Relieve Stress And Promote Relaxation

By Amy Joyson

I0412118

by the trademark owner. All trademarks and brands within this book are for clarifying purposes only and are the owned by the owners themselves, not affiliated with this document.

Disclaimer – Please read!

The information provided in this book is designed to provide helpful information on the subjects discussed. This book is not meant to be used, nor should it be used, to diagnose or treat any medical condition. For diagnosis or treatment of any medical problem, consult your own physician. The publisher and author are not responsible for any specific health or allergy needs that may require medical supervision and are not liable for any damages or negative consequences from any treatment, action, application or preparation, to any person reading or following the information in this book. References are provided for informational purposes only and do not constitute endorsement of any websites or other sources. Readers should be aware that the websites listed in this book may change.

Table of Contents

Introduction

When it comes to administering essential oils for their amazing health benefits, few techniques are as effective or complementary as massage. Not only does massage address the practical need for introducing essential oils to the body, but also brings a whole host of therapeutic benefits to the table in its own right. Simply when used on their own, the unique remedial properties of essential oils can offer a wide number of health benefits, from the alleviation of pain, stress or tension, to boosting circulation and energy. When used in combination with the art of massage, the curative effect of these substances can be multiplied manifold. This book will explore the powerful link between essential oils and massage, and provide some guidelines as to how the two can be used in marriage to create a truly holistic form of therapy.

As many readers of this guide will be aware, the previous book in my aromatherapy series provided an introductory overview of essential oils and their therapeutic potential. While this first guide was designed as a basic 'primer' on the various properties and applications of different essential oils, this book will take a deeper and more nuanced look at the role of massage in aromatherapy. Although this guide has been written in a way that makes it accessible to those without prior knowledge of aromatherapy, it is highly recommended that those who have not yet done so take some time to explore the first book in this series to enhance their aromatherapy education. Find out how to find it on the last pages of this book! The aim of this book is to help you to safely and conscientiously begin exploring the wonderful marriage of massage and aromatherapy, providing some useful and interesting background, while also showcasing some specific tips and techniques for remedying a wide range of complaints and ailments. By the end of this guide you should feel empowered to effectively combine the complementary arts of massage and aromatherapy to treat a wide range of conditions.

This book is broken down into ten chapters, each with a different focus when it comes to aromatherapy and massage. The beginning of the guide will cover some 'getting started' basics, and provide an overview on the link between massage and essential oils. The latter half of the book, meanwhile, will look at some applications of massage and aromatherapy for specialized treatments. Chapter one will take a look at the fundamentals of massage and essential oils, exploring the history of the combination of the two in holistic treatment, the benefits of massage when it comes to aromatherapy (and of massage in its own right), and some of the advantages that massage has as a delivery method over other types of aromatherapy treatments. Chapter two will take a brief but essential look at the issue of safety when it comes to delivering essential oils through massage. This will cover the importance of diluting essential oils in carrier oils (which I discussed in some detail in my first book), as well as some general tips when it comes to safe practice regarding both essential oils and massage.

Chapter three will take an overview look at various massage techniques that can be used to administer essential oils for therapeutic purposes. This will include an exploration of techniques that can be used for massage therapy in their own right (i.e. independent of aromatherapy), as well as those that have been specifically developed as a complement to the practice of aromatherapy. Finally, chapters four through nine will discuss the different targeted treatments that can be carried out using massage and essential oils, with each chapter having a different focus. For example, chapter five will look at stress relief; chapter six will cover pain relief etc. Included in each of these chapters will be an overview of the essential oils that can be useful for each targeted treatment, aromatherapy blends that can be made in to targeted recipes and tinctures, and the massage techniques that will be most suitable for that particular treatment.

In summary, this guide will provide newcomers to the world of aromatherapy with a range of skills and applications that can be delivered both generally, and for a range of specific conditions. By the end of this book, readers will hopefully be armed with the knowledge to confidently explore the union between aromatherapy and massage, and to develop their interest in the wonderful world of essential oils in earnest.

Chapter 1 – Massage and essential oils

The History of Massage and Essential Oils

Massage and essential oils have long been paired in a powerful therapeutic union across many different cultures and eras. Essential oils have been referenced in many an ancient text as being imbued with divine, spiritual properties. These oils were often manifested in the shape of sacred tinctures or holy balms which were in many instances applied to a person with what today could be considered the most rudimentary form of massage. Indeed, when one considers the origins of massage, the practice holds a similar place in history as do these revered oils– as part of the foundation of sacred ritual. Ayurvedic Indians and Chinese Buddhists alike practiced massage as one method aimed at manipulating the most base and carnal representation of the self – the 'flesh' – to a more revered and pure spiritual plane. For centuries, massage was largely associated with this act of ritual and any tangible physical benefit was largely thought to be a side effect of spiritual healing. The Ayurvedic view, for example, holds that an illness or pathology is incurred by an individual when they fall out of spiritual harmony with the world around them. Traditionally, massage was one way of recalibrating this misalignment, providing both spiritual and physical reparation.

The practice of massage itself is estimated to date back at least some 5,000 years, to the ancient civilizations of Asia and the Middle East. Though it is uncertain when the union between massage and essential oils first occurred, the Ancient Egyptians made some of the earliest forays in this area. The Egyptians were renowned for their topical use of essential oils, which they applied through a range of applications – from embalming, to cosmetics, to massage. The practice of utilizing essential oils with massage was also followed by other contemporary apothecaries of the ancient world, including those of Indian and Chinese cultures. Later, during the first millennium BCE, the Eastern practice of massage migrated to the West; first, to Greece, to complement that civilizations penchant for athletics and pursuit of therapeutic medicine; and later, to Rome. There, physicians honed the arts of massage, adopted from their Hellenistic neighbors and turned it into an intractable part of civic life. Wealthy citizens of Rome regularly received massages from doctors and other trained professionals who delivered such services both at public baths and private residences. These treatments were typically used to deliver various exotic oils which were applied deliberately for their medicinal and cosmetic properties.

Over the following centuries, massage lost its appeal among Western cultures, only to be rekindled during the 19th century. This renaissance came when Swedish physician Per Henrik Ling developed a massage treatment program specifically for gymnasts, to encourage flexibility and recovery. Later, during the early 20th century, a 'rebirth' also occurred in the field of aromatherapy, as the work of French chemist René Gattefossé invigorated interest in the ancient practice. Perhaps inspired by these two movements, one of the first aromatherapy practitioners in modern times to marry these complementary fields was Austrian born Madame Marguerite Maury. Following the death of her young child, husband and father, Maury undertook training as a nurse and moved to France. There she dedicated herself to the study of aromatherapy, in particular the application of essential oils via massage. Later, she was responsible for opening the earliest aromatherapy clinics in Great Britain, France and Switzerland, which occurred by the mid-20th century. During the second half of the century, the practice of applying essential oils through massage had become commonplace, as Westerners began to turn away from traditional medicine and towards 'alternative' remedies for the treatment and prevention of illness. Though much of the encyclopedic collective knowledge that comprises contemporary massage and aromatherapy is heavily rooted in ancient techniques and practice, it has nonetheless evolved into a highly studied alternative to traditional Western methods of treating illness.

Today, massage and aromatherapy are inextricably intertwined, and this method of application remains one of the most popular for delivering the remedial benefits of essential oils. From the above we can see that it is only very recently that the highly scientific and physiological practice of massage as we know it has come into being. However, as a therapeutic treatment, massage still inhabits the strange space between the oft derided mass of 'alternative therapy', and the more rigorously scientific and cautious school of 'Western medicine'. Despite this, the fact that massage and aromatherapy have been used across millennia to the present day serves well to highlight the power of this therapeutic union.

The therapeutic benefits of massage

When practiced independently of other treatments, massage can have an enormous range of therapeutic benefits, let alone when used as a method for administering essential oils. The first and perhaps most well-known of these benefits, is the ability for massage to relieve pain and tension through the direct stimulation and manipulation of individual muscle fibers. While this has perhaps been one of the main appeals of massage during its long history of practice, it has only relatively recently become understood why the act of massage can provide therapeutic relief in this way. While previously it was understood that a muscular complaint that led to a bad back may have been the result of either a weighted conscious or spiritual affliction, we know today that this type of pathology is in fact caused by a muscular or skeletal problem. By using massage – that is, kneading, prodding, chopping and manipulating the flesh – these pathologies can be put right by hand.

However, there are a range of other surprising health benefits when it comes to the power of massage. For example, massage can also aid in improving our overall mood, by soothing anxiety and depression. The human touch is an incredibly important component in our overall wellbeing. Not only is this a basic human emotional need, but has also proven to have some incredible physiological effects on proper hormonal function. Studies have indicated that infants that have been deprived of human contact have elevated levels of the stress hormone, cortisol, in their bloodstreams, as well as lowered levels of oxytocin and vasopressin which are essential when it comes to emotional and social bonding, as well as healthy physiological function. This cocktail of hormones and neurotransmitters circulate through our blood vessels and are the very drivers of much of our psychological and emotional being, are thus heavily regulated by human contact. Interestingly, this touch doesn't even have to be delivered by a family member, friend or lover; even the humble hands of an unknown masseuse can be enough to stir up the tempest of chemicals within, and make us know what it is to really feel *human.*

How massage enhances aromatherapy

Massage has many distinct advantages compared to other methods of essential oil application, not least of which are the independent benefits that one may acquire from massage. To understand why massage can be such an effective method for delivering essential oils, we first need to take a quick recap regarding how essential oils work in our bodies. There are three main ways that essential oils can enter the body: through ingestion, inhalation or absorption through the skin. The first of these methods is perhaps the least common, given that it can lead to a patient experiencing the most adverse effects. Though some essential oils are quite mild and are generally safe to be ingested, many are rather potent and can lead to irritation of the digestive system.

Furthermore, some essential oils can be toxic when ingested. For these reasons, internal use of essential oils is rare, and is generally only practiced under the supervision or instruction of a trained professional. Leaving aside ingestion, we are left with the two methods of inhalation and topical application. In the case of the former, the perfume of essential oils stimulates the brain's limbic system, which influences much of the physiological response throughout the body. For example, it is believed to affect things such as adrenal function, emotion, memory and general behavior. The introduction of essential oils, meanwhile, can have a profound effect in influencing the function of the limbic system, and thus have a significant carry over effect into these areas of bodily function. Finally, the application of essential oils to the skin is thought to be particularly effective in treating both conditions relating to blood flow, as well as complaints that are localized to the area of treatment. Due to their extremely fine molecular composition, essential oils are typically easily absorbed into the bloodstream through the skin.

In addition to the dermal absorption and inhalation that typically occurs during a massage treatment that incorporates aromatherapy, massage can also boost circulation (which can enhance the uptake of essential oils into the blood stream), encourage proper function of the body's lymphatic system, and work with the active properties of essential oils to engage and invigorate the mind. All of these benefits (and more) will be discussed in detail in later chapters.

Chapter 2 – Safety

When it comes to the application of any kind of therapeutic remedy – from aromatherapy, to massage, to the administration of pharmaceuticals – safety precautions should always be observed during treatment. Furthermore, as with the overall application of essential oils for therapeutic purposes, it is important to keep certain safety precautions in mind when applying essential oils through massage. Due to aromatherapy's status as an 'alternative' remedy, the potential potency of volatile ingredients used in its practice are often not treated with the respect and caution that they deserve. Likewise, massage is often attempted by amateur enthusiasts who can do real damage if certain precautions are not observed. This chapter will explore some of the key considerations to follow to ensure the safe practice of aromatherapy massage, both in terms of massage and essential oils in their own right.

Irritation, Sensitization and Photosensitivity

It is extremely important for amateur aromatherapists to avoid using essential oils in certain situations where an adverse reaction to an oil may occur. Though many of these incredible natural compounds exhibit powerful and fascinating remedial properties, the very active ingredients that give these oils their potency and therapeutic qualities can also induce a negative reaction in some individuals. When it comes to the topical application of essential oils, there are three types of reaction that one should be aware of: *irritation, sensitization* and *photosensitivity*. There are several essential oils that may cause severe skin irritation in some patients and, as such, should be used with some caution. These include, for example, peppermint, clove and cinnamon. This is by no means an exhaustive list as there are dozens upon dozens of essential oils that are in common use for aromatherapy and each can induce a different effect depending on the individual. Although many are deemed 'safe' essential oils (such as lavender or chamomile) with very little chance of inducing an adverse reaction, every essential oil should be treated with the same level of caution. Symptoms of skin irritation can involve a rash, redness or inflammation around the treated area, and can vary in terms of the level of severity. Normally, irritation induced by essential oils is minor and will resolve itself within 24 to 48 hours of exposure to the irritant. However, in some (more extreme) cases of allergic reaction, irritation may result in severe burns and require medical treatment.

There are a number of oils which may lead to what is known as 'sensitization' of a patient, which involves an immune system reaction to an aromatherapy treatment. When sensitization occurs via massage, typically there is evidence of a local reaction; however, sensitization is normally characterized by a more acute and general immune system response. This is generally exhibited by the manifestation of symptoms that can seem unrelated to the treatment or the treatment area (as opposed to irritation, which is typified by a localized reaction). This can be seen, for example, in the appearance of a general rash or eczema throughout the body after an aromatherapy massage treatment. Ways to avoid sensitization reactions include: testing oils in small concentrations when patients have not previously been exposed to that particular oil; using essential oils that are high in aldehydes and phenols with caution; and ensuring that essential oils are *never* applied neat unless otherwise advised by a trained aromatherapy professional. Once sensitization to a particular oil has occurred this is normally permanent, so it is important to take steps to prevent this reaction from occurring in the first instance.

Another way in which a patient can react negatively to an essential oil treatment is through what is known as chemically induced photosensitivity. Certain essential oils contain compounds that can cause increased sensitivity to UV light, such as that emitted by the sun. These oils are classified as *phototoxic*, and can lead a patient to experience severe burns following exposure to the sun. Some essential oils that may induce photosensitivity include bergamot, lemon, lime and any other citrus derived compounds (this shared characteristic among the citrus family is due to the presence of high aldehyde concentrations associated with oils in this group). To avoid photosensitivity, patients should avoid contact with direct sunlight for up to 12 hours after receiving a treatment with oils that exhibit phototoxic properties. Additionally, the chances of a phototoxic reaction can be limited if this oils are used exclusively in well-diluted concentrations.

Fortunately, there are some steps that can be taken to reduce the general risk of an adverse episode during topical exposure to essential oils. First, it is *always* advised that essential oils be used in diluted concentrations before being directly introduced to the body. When applying essential oils through massage, this involves making a 'blend' by mixing the active essential oil with a more chemically inert 'carrier oil'. Carrier oils are typically derived from plant matter and are comprised of essential fatty acids (EFAs) and other stable compounds that do not interact in a volatile way with the skin. The great thing about these carrier oils is that they are also often rich in vitamins and other nutrients which can enhance a massage blend's therapeutic effect, and what's more, are typically very beneficial for the skin. The physical properties of these carrier oils also offer a lot more lubrication which can make a massage more pleasant for the recipient. Using carrier oils to create massage blends will be discussed in more detail in chapter four.

High risk groups

When conducting *any* type of aromatherapy treatment that involves essential oils, it is very important to recall that certain groups may be more vulnerable to experiencing adverse events than others. One should avoid using essential oils with children for a few key precautions. First, kids are more likely to experience a sensitization reaction from essential oils due to their smaller overall body mass and the higher effect that normal concentrations can have on their physiologies. Essential oils should generally be precluded from use in children under 12 unless otherwise indicate by a trained aromatherapist. Second, the elderly can also be more vulnerable to an adverse reaction from essential oils and care should be taken in practicing any form of aromatherapy with this demographic. Next, one should be careful to screen patients for potential complications due to pre-existing medical conditions. This is because particular essential oils can induce adverse physiological reactions, to which some with certain conditions may be more vulnerable. For example, certain essential oils are classified as *hepatoxic* and can cause liver damage in high concentrations, to which those with pre-existing liver disease may be more vulnerable. Finally, essential oils should be used with caution in pregnant women as not enough research has been conducted into the effect of aromatherapy treatments on fetal development. It is safe to presume that any treatment received by the mother will have some residual effect on the baby that she is carrying. What's more, some essential oils are contraindicated for use in pregnant women as they are classified as *abortifacients* and may induce labor in expectant women.

Safety with massage

Having covered a few of the basic safety tips when it comes to using essential oils in their own right, we will now turn to the art of massage and consider some of the necessary precautions for the safe practice of this therapeutic treatment. Because it is not invasive, massage is one of the safer therapeutic treatments around. There is generally a negligible or non-existent risk for things like infection or pharmacokinetic reaction that may be associated with other treatments. However, that is not to say that massage is without risk. All good masseurs should be aware of the potential for harm to be done to a patient through massage, while being sensitive of some measures that can be taken to minimize the risk of injury. The most obvious way in which a patient can be harmed through massage is the event of first or second degree muscle damage. A first degree, or mild strain, is the most likely injury to occur during massage and may happen as a result of improper manipulation of muscle tissue. Second degree (or moderate) strains are more likely to occur when a muscle injury is exacerbated by an overly vigorous massage. Third degree strain (severe muscle or ligament damage) as a result of massage therapy is rather unlikely, although possible in very few cases (normally where a second degree strain has already occurred). The most important thing to be aware of when delivering a massage is whether the patient has any existing injuries that could be potentially made worse through a very firm massage. Additionally, it is also vital that a masseur monitors their patient and looks for signs of discomfort during the treatment. While a firm massage can often deliver the best therapeutic results, amateur masseurs should be careful to not overdo it when it comes to applied pressure and should be sure to ease up if there is any indication that a massage might be hurting a patient. Extremely rough massage may result in bruising or minor nerve or muscle damage and should be avoided.

Although injury through massage is rare, it is important to be aware of conditions or characteristics that may make massage an unsuitable treatment option. For example, the elderly and frail, and young children and infants should generally not be treated with massage as their bodily tissues can be more delicate and prone to injury. Additionally, those in a physical state that makes them more prone to injury should avoid receiving massage therapy. This can include those who have recently received surgery, have open wounds or sores in or around the treatment area, or have a history of blood clotting disorders, such as deep vein thrombosis. Additionally, massage is contraindicated in patients with fever as the action of massage may exacerbate symptoms and make the subject feel worse. Massage should also be avoided in patients who have communicable diseases, as these may in some cases be transferred to the masseur, or to subsequent patients.

When practicing aromatherapy via massage, most adverse incidents can be avoided by exercising common sense. By never using undiluted essential oils in a massage, limiting treatment in the abovementioned higher risk groups, and communicating with your patient to ensure that they let you know as soon as something doesn't 'feel right', you can be confident about delivering massage therapy in the most safe and productive way possible. With these safety basics covered, let's now move on to an introduction to fundamental massage techniques.

Chapter 3 – Massage techniques

There are a number of massage techniques that all can be used to treat a range of conditions and improve general wellbeing, especially when combined with aromatherapy. At its most basic, massage is a way of introducing essential oils into the skin until they are absorbed into the bloodstream through the pores – a chemical process known as *osmosis*. The volatile compounds found in the oils are then circulated throughout the body's various systems and tissues, typically resulting in a net therapeutic effect. While massage can simply be looked at a rudimentary means of physically effecting this reaction, it can be (and usually is) so much more than this. For example, massage, as discussed above, is a great way to complement aromatherapy treatments with added perks like improved circulation, relaxation and hormonal release. In fact, there are a wide range of different massage techniques that can be applied to induce different physiological effects based on the desired outcome of treatment. Some of these advanced techniques will be discussed in later chapters. In this chapter, however, we will introduce some basic and necessary massage concepts that can be used in conjunction with most aromatherapy treatments.

Those of you familiar with the first book in this series will recall being introduced to some basic massage concepts and terminology. We will now recount this introduction and expand on the information found therein by providing a more detailed account on how and why it is important to master these massage techniques. At its most basic, massage involves manipulating and kneading the flesh of any part of the body to induce a feeling of greater ultimate comfort in the recipient. It is, in essence, a simple enough concept that just about anyone can be asked to deliver a massage or 'back rub' and go on to do so with a reasonable degree of efficacy. Typically, however, any uneducated attempts at massage, while beneficial for inducing a general sense of relaxation and stress relief, can be hit and miss when it comes to delivering a specified therapeutic treatment. To get to this level, one must *learn* the art of massage, including all of the individual components and techniques that go into delivering a successful massage treatment. We can think about massage in this way as similar the act of hitting a golf ball. Most people, when asked to strike a golf ball with a golf club, will be able to do so, some with greater skill or finesse than others. As a rule, however, it is those who are aware of what goes into the art of constructing a 'perfect' golf swing that will be able to drive the ball furthest and fairest. Additionally, those who have the opportunity to practice their swing more regularly will typically become more proficient in striking the ball in a true and correct way. The same can be said for massage; those who are armed with knowledge and technique, and have had the opportunity to hone their craft, will be much more likely to achieve their treatment goal than those who are not armed with such knowledge. With this in mind, we will now take a look at some of the most important basic massage concepts, including a discussion of their intended function. (We will focus in this chapter on many of the techniques that comprise Swedish massage, as this is perhaps the most well-known form of massage in practice today, and thus, the simplest to demonstrate through written instruction).

One of the simplest and most important ways to begin a massage treatment is with a technique known as *effleurage*. This method, which literally means 'to skim the surface', involves exactly that – stroking the flesh of a subject with the fingertips in broad, circular movements. This technique serves a number of purposes. First, it induces a sense of relaxation in the patient which can be the goal of a massage treatment in and of itself, or can prove complementary to other desired outcomes. Second, effleurage encourages blood flow in the local area, which can encourage healing, and make aromatherapy treatment more effective as essential oils are more easily drawn into and distributed throughout the body when circulation is improved. When practicing the effleurage technique, it is important to remember to initially use long, light strokes. Additionally, it is important to begin contact with the fingertips and to smoothly transition to a flat palm. The emphasis on applied pressure should be placed on the upward stroke, with the return lightly skimming across the skin. *Deep effleurage* can involve using firmer pressure on the skin and can be effective in treating muscular pain. Effleurage is a great way to begin a massage as it not only helps a patient to relax by using gentle, repetitive motions, but is also an effective way to introduce massage oils or products evenly to the skin.

Another important fundamental massage technique is what is known as *petrissage*. Also known as kneading, this technique involves firmly pressing the flesh and manipulating muscle tissue with the fingers, thumbs, palms or knuckles. This technique generally focuses intently on one particular area of the body, and can be an effective way of alleviating tension in a specific area. When practicing petrissage, movements should be slow, deliberate and rhythmical. Intense pressure should be avoided, although the general technique should be firm.

Tapotement (derived from the French for 'to tap or drum') is yet another core massage technique, and involves drumming the skin in a percussive manner to encourage blood flow and stimulate nervous system response. It is typically administered using a cupped hand or the tips of the fingers, and has five main variations: 'beating' (using a closed fist), 'slapping' (with the palm side of the fingers), 'hacking' (a chopping motion using the straight edge of the hand), 'tapping' (with the fingertips) or 'cupping' (by shaping the hand into a cup shape and gently striking the target area). For all of the above variations of tapotement, the standard technique typically involves rapid, soft blows from alternating hands.

While the above takes into account some of the more basic methods for delivering massage therapy, we will explore some more advanced techniques that can complement your aromatherapy treatments in later chapters. These include the *raindrop technique, Indian head massage* and *lymphatic massage.*

Chapter 4 – Essential oil blends for massage

As discussed above in our earlier chapter on safety, essential oils should generally never be applied to the skin 'neat' or undiluted. In order to avoid this, essential oils are typically combined with a larger quantity of a given carrier oil which not only makes the delivery of aromatherapy through massage safer, but also provides for a more pleasant massage experience. We will now take a look at everything you need to know about creating aromatherapy blends for massage, including the different types of carrier oils that can be used to create blends and their properties, suggestions on how to buy and choose the right carrier oil for your blends, and some advice on how to properly prepare and store blends.

Carrier oil basics

Those who read our introductory book will recall that we covered a few basics when it comes to carrier oils and their properties. This section will take the basics already covered and expand on them in greater detail to arm you with even greater knowledge on this subject. To recap, carrier oils are typically derived from nuts, seeds or kernels and are primarily comprised of various essential fatty acids (EFAs), as well as other important and vital nutrients. Carrier oils are in fact much more deserving of being labelled as 'oils' than are essential oils; the former are lipids, while the later can be described as aromatic hydrocarbons. Essential oils mix well with carrier oils because the former are what is known as *lipophilic* – that is, they are chemically attracted to lipids and naturally emulsify when combined with oils. This makes carrier oils and essential oils great partners to combine in blends for use during massage. Not only do the two mix well, but the remedial properties of essential oils can be well complemented by the nutrients found within carrier oils.

25

Furthermore, carrier oils provide a great lubricating consistency for a massage-friendly aid.

There are a hundreds, if not thousands of different prefabricated proprietary blends available for purchase from various vendors of essential oil related products. These are typically made from specially formulated recipes that have been designed to treat very specific complaints or ailments. These blends can be great for newcomers to the world of essential oils, as well as those who don't want to deal with the hassle of making their own blends and don't mind spending a bit more money doing so. However, there are a few reasons why it can be a good idea to branch out and create your own blends using individual essential and carrier oils. First, although it can be a bit of an effort to set everything up from scratch, using your own range of basic supplies to create massage blends offers a lot more versatility in terms the possible combinations and permutations of ingredients. You may personally find, for example, that you prefer using one essential oil over another when the two exhibit similar properties – a freedom that isn't afforded when using proprietary blends. Secondly, creating your own blends at home will actually lead you to learn a lot more about the distinct properties of different essential oils and become a better aromatherapist in the process. When you buy a prefabricated blend for 'stress relief' off the shelf, it can be easy to use this and not actively think about *why* the blend is good for stress. But if one is to make their own recipe from scratch, using careful measures of specially chosen essential oils and combining them with a suitably chosen carrier oil, this can in itself be a valuable educative experience. Instead of learning that a proprietary blend for stress relief is a good application for stress relief, one will soon learn that lavender and chamomile (for example) are the true heroes when it comes to inducing calm in a patient. Third, when you use proprietary blends it can be difficult to guarantee the quality of the product you are using. Although there are many reputable vendors offering high quality proprietary blends, there is always a risk that they may contain lower quality ingredients than if formulated from scratch at home. Fourth and finally, making your own blends is definitely more economical in the long run. This is especially true if you plan on committing to practicing aromatherapy for the long term, as individual ingredients work out a lot cheaper than when purchased in a combined form. Essential oils generally have an indefinite shelf life, and while carrier oils can go rancid after a while, you will still work out better off if you plan on using the oils on a regular basis.

When it comes to choosing the right carrier oil for the right massage application, there are a few key things to consider. First, different oils can have vastly different properties that make them largely unsuitable to use as the main oil in a massage blend. For example, avocado or wheatgerm oils can provide great benefits when used in a blend thanks to the array of vitamins and nutrients they contain; however, their viscosity, strong odor and expense typically precludes them from being suitable as the main carrier in a blend. Instead, it is often a good idea to mix a small concentration of these oils (20 percent or so) with a cheaper, more neutral oil (such as grapeseed) to still enjoy the benefits they can offer to a massage blend.

Choosing the right carrier oil(s)

With this in mind, given that there are dozens upon dozens of potential carrier oils that may be used and combined in a blend in different ratios, how exactly does one choose the right ones for a given blend? As a rule, it is a good idea when starting out to keep it simple and limit the number of carrier oils in your selection. Not only will this prove more manageable for a beginner, but can also prevent wastage from occurring as some carrier oils can go bad when stored for too long. With this in mind, there are a few key pointers for choosing your 'core collection' of carrier oils when getting started with aromatherapy massage. As mentioned above, carrier oils fall into primary and secondary categories. Primary carrier oils are those that make up the majority of a blend, and typically exhibit more neutral or 'lighter' characteristics than secondary carriers. They are also often less expensive products and make their use as the primary constituent of a blend a sensible option. These can include, for example, grapeseed oil, canola oil, olive oil and coconut oil. Secondary carrier oils are those that may exhibit more unique characteristics, but which would overpower a blend with a strong odor or prove too expensive for use on their own. It is generally a good idea to have a couple of different carrier oils that fall into each of these categories.

Another important distinction between various carrier oils is their consistency. This is clearly an important consideration when it comes to massage, as massage therapy is a highly tactile experience. The consistency of a carrier oil at room temperature can vary wildly from liquid (e.g. olive or grapeseed oil), to soft solid (e.g. coconut oil or shea butter), to brittle solid (e.g. cocoa or illipe butter). Within these variations there are also other subtleties to take into consideration, such as texture (the stickiness of shea butter versus the oiliness of coconut oil, for example), rate of absorption (a very important consideration in therapeutic massage depending on the intended treatment), and odor (neutral, as in grapeseed oil, or aromatic, as in coconut oil). Meanwhile, another great characteristic of some carrier oils is their ability to act as a preservative in blends containing other oils which have a short shelf life. For example, grapeseed oil has a relatively short shelf life of about a year, but when combined with a small quantity of wheatgerm oil can last significantly longer than this. Because of the multitude of variations that can occur between different carrier oils, it is a good idea to try and build up a collection of a few that offer the biggest degree of difference and will allow you to experiment with their different properties. Which carrier oils you choose to make part of your core collection can be a highly subjective and personal choice; however, for those too overwhelmed by choice and unsure where to start, a good core collection might involve the following:

Grapeseed oil: this is a good base oil that can be used in many different combinations. It has a neutral odor and light, oily texture, and is a liquid oil at room temperature. Grapeseed oil has a shelf life of a little under 12 months.

Coconut oil: unrefined coconut oil is a wonderful soft solid carrier that is solid at room temperature, but quickly melts to an oily consistency when applied to the body. This oil is very fragrant, and rich in essential minerals and nutrients. Coconut oil has a shelf life of a little under 12 months.

Jojoba oil: technically a liquid wax rather than an oil, jojoba is liquid at room temperature and absorbs into the skin relatively well. It is also rich in vitamin E, making it a good treatment for cosmetic applications. Jojoba is very stable and has a long shelf life, and may be used to extend the shelf life of other carrier oils.

Avocado oil: this oil, thanks to containing a high concentration of vitamins and fatty acids, is very nourishing and soothing for the skin. However, it is also a very sticky, waxy oil and will leave an oily film on the skin. For this reason, it is best used a small quantities as the secondary carrier oil in a blend. Avocado oil has a shelf life of between 6 to 12 months.

Shea butter: this can be a good main constituent for making 'body butters' which make for versatile massage treatments. Shea butter is very soft at room temperature, and has a waxy, slightly tacky consistency when applied to the skin. It also has a pleasant odor, however, this may overwhelm other carriers in the same blend. Shea butter can be a good agent for making topical creams and balms and has a very good shelf life of up to 24 months.

With these few carrier oils/butters in your core collection, you will find that you will have enough options on hand to formulate suitable blends for a number of treatments. Of course, this just scratches the surface and there are many, many more different carrier oils available that can offer a range of unique, nourishing properties for different treatments. For that reason, I encourage you to keep exploring what different carrier oils can offer as your interest in aromatherapy develops over time.

This concludes our introduction to massage and aromatherapy. You are now armed with the most basic of knowledge when it comes to how and why the two disciplines make for a great combination. The remaining chapters in this book will explore treatments for specific purposes, and will introduce a few new concepts along the way.

Chapter 4 –Stress relief

Stress is one of the most debilitating and prolific health risks in society today. There is a proven and commonly accepted link between stress and poor health, yet many of us accept stress as just a part of our everyday lives. Our fast paced, high stakes, 'always on' world means that there is little (if any!) down time in many people's day-to-day schedules. Sadly, it is not an uncommon experience to feel as though you are holding on by your fingernails as life whips around you, while telling yourself that the one or two weeks of holiday planned in the distant future will be enough to keep you sane for another year. Fortunately, even though we may not be able to do a lot to change the things causing stress in our lives, we can take some steps to minimize the natural stress response of our bodies. There is perhaps no better way to calm one's nerves and elevated stress levels, than with a long, relaxing massage. As mentioned above, human touch can be highly effective in making us feel calm, a fact which is made possible through the hormonal chemistry of the human body. Prolonged touch between two people has been shown stimulate the release of the bonding chemical, oxytocin. This hormone is released in high doses through events in which human contact typically occurs, including hugging, kissing, sex and even light touch between two people. Most interestingly, at least when it comes to controlling our stress levels, oxytocin has been shown to have a *suppressant* effect on the body's stress hormone, cortisol. So that means that the more we expose ourselves to physical interactions with other people, the less cortisol induced stress we are likely to feel. When the stress relieving properties of certain essential oils are added into the mix, massage can provide a much needed reprieve for even the most cortisol stricken individuals. We'll now take a look at some of the most effective oils, blends and treatments for stress relief through the combination of aromatherapy and massage.

One of the best essential oils for inducing feelings of calm is lavender. Lavender is great for a whole range of therapeutic conditions – in fact, it is an absolutely *essential* essential oil. There are lots of essential oils that have loads of excellent and varied remedial properties, however, lavender is really queen when it comes to the world of aromatherapy. It is wonderfully versatile and can be applied for a range of purposes: from disinfecting wounds, to burns treatment, to pain relief. It is also one of the very few essential oils that can safely be applied to the skin 'neat' or undiluted. In summary, if you had to choose a 'desert island' essential oil, lavender should naturally be the go to option! Not least among the valued properties of lavender, is its ability to be utilized as an effective treatment for stress relief. Thanks to the versatility of lavender, we'll talk more about this special oil later on, but for now it is important to remember – *lavender is great for inducing a sense of calm.* Clary sage is another essential oil that has a particularly good effect in calming a patient's nerves. Derived from the steam distilled buds and leaves of the Clary Sage plant (*Salvea Sclarea),* this essential oil exhibits many parallel and complementary properties to lavender, especially when it comes to inducing a calmative effect. This remarkable herb has long been valued in its own right for its many and varied medicinal qualities, including its effect as an antidepressant, sedative and nervine agent. Care should be taken when using clary sage in combination with alcohol, as the herb can intensify the effects of this drug. Finally, geranium oil has been shown to be a highly effective emotional 'balancing' agent, which can greatly assist those suffering from anxiety or depression.

With the above calm inducing essential oils in mind, we'll now take a look at how to combine these into a great massage blend for stress relief. When making a blend for stress relief, it is perfectly acceptable to use a fairly neutral carrier oil, such as grapeseed as the primary constituent. This is because the essential oils are really doing the lion's share of the work here, and work in two distinct ways to create a feeling of calm. First, the scent of the essential oils works through the body's olfactory system to stimulate the limbic system, and helps to regulate impulses from the central nervous system that lead to an overactive adrenal response. For this reason, a carrier oil with a relatively neutral scent should be used here. The volatile compounds of the active essential oils also work by entering the body through the bloodstream; from here, they circulate throughout the body where they can relax muscles and also influence cortisol and adrenaline levels in the body by limiting overactive stress hormone production. As such, opting for a carrier oil with a moderately good rate of absorption (such as grapeseed or apricot kernel oils) is recommended.

With this in mind, the following treatment makes for a good remedy when treating stress in a patient: 3 drops of clary sage oil; 3 drops of lavender oil; 3 drops of geranium oil; 10mL grapeseed oil. All ingredients should be combined in a dark glass jar and shaken to combine. When applying via massage, the applicant should take a small amount of the blend (about the size of a dime) and rub together in their palms to warm before applying to the patient. Focus the massage on the back and shoulders, which can carry a lot of tension in a person experiencing high levels of stress. If you have more time, a full body massage can provide great benefits to a patient suffering from stress. Apply the same technique to the legs, arms, back, neck, shoulders, feet, hands and head. A comprehensive massage such as this (which can take around 45 minutes to an hour) can ensure the complete relaxation of the recipient as they become fully immersed in the experience. Good results can also be achieved using what is known as the *raindrop technique* which will be discussed further in the later chapter on meditation.

Chapter 5 – Pain relief

As mentioned earlier, massage therapy itself is perhaps most typically associated with the providing direct pain relief from sore muscles. Whether this is the muscular pain felt from a sports strain or discomfort caused by sleeping in a contorted position, a vigorous massage is often the key to relieving discomfort. When combined with aromatherapy treatment, however, massage takes on a whole new dimension of pain relief potential. Used in this way, aromatherapy can be the key to not only successfully treating local muscular pain, but can also yield positive results when attempting to relieve pain felt throughout the body. The following chapter will look at various strategies for treating pain through aromatherapy and massage, with a spotlight on the wonderful pain relief properties of lavender oil.

Already discussed in the previous chapter of this book, lavender exhibits some remarkable properties which make it a highly versatile essential oil. Among lavender oil's long list of remedial effects is its potential as an agent for pain relief. It is particularly effective when it comes to relieving inflammation and is useful for treating local soft tissue pain that may be caused by swelling. Additionally, lavender can act as a muscle relaxant and can provide effective relief from the pain associated with muscle spasm. Another great essential oil when it comes to pain relief is chamomile. Like lavender, chamomile is also a very gentle essential oil and can be used neat (although should only be done so under advice or supervision of a trained professional). Chamomile has two main varieties that are widely used in aromatherapy: Roman (*Anthemis nobilis*) and German (*Matricaria chamomilla*) Chamomile. The latter has strong anti-inflammatory properties and is generally the best choice when it comes to pain relief. Another powerful essential oil with strong pain relief potential is rosemary. Rosemary's power also lies in its ability to reduce inflammation, and like lavender and chamomile, also has a strong calmative effect which can act to mitigate the brain's pain response. There are a number of other essential oils which can provide pain relief and can be used in combination with a massage treatment. These include peppermint, helichrysum, eucalyptus, clove bud, basil and marjoram, among many others.

When choosing a carrier oil for use in a pain relief massage blend, borage seed oil can be a good choice. This is an especially good carrier oil when it comes to treating pain and inflammation associated with rheumatological diseases, such as arthritis or gout. Again, like the abovementioned essential oils, this oil has the effect of targeting soft tissue inflammation which can help to reduce tenderness, soreness and swelling. Please note, however, that the application of barrage seed oil should be avoided in those with a predisposition to liver conditions, as the carrier contains *hepatoxic* properties which can cause liver failure in extreme situations. This oil is also contraindicated for use in pregnant women as it can act as an *emmengogue* which may stimulate labor at any stage of a pregnancy. When these factors are a concern, a more neutral carrier oil can prove to be a safer choice; however, it is important to remember that patients falling into such 'high risk' categories should be cleared for treatment by a physician before any course of massage or aromatherapy is undertaken.

When applying massage for pain relief, the massage should above all use gentle strokes and light pressure in the affected area. More pressure can be applied if it is suspected that the pain is due to muscular tension or 'knots'. However, if the recipient indicates that the massage is causing any additional pain, the treatment should be paused. If the patient indicates that the increase in pain has abated, the massage may continue; however, if pain levels remain elevated, treatment should be halted. (*Please note, this is a good general practice to apply to all massage treatments, not only those in which the treatment of pain is a concern*).

Chapter 6 –Treating chronic illness

For those suffering with chronic illness of almost any kind, gentle massage can be a highly effective way to administer essential oils for their healing properties, and to enjoy the positive effects that massage can have on our health. Many, many different conditions may be treated and symptoms alleviated through the use of aromatherapy and massage, but for the sake of simplicity, we will only examine two in this chapter. Chronic fatigue syndrome (CFS) is one such condition whose symptoms may be alleviated through aromatherapy massage. As the name suggests, this illness is associated with constant feelings of tiredness, and general sluggishness and malaise. Although there is no official diagnosis for CFS, there is anecdotal evidence that suggests that the condition afflicts thousands of people. It is normally indicated in patients after an acute viral illness, such as the Ross River or herpes viruses. Fibromyalgia, is another condition associated with severe chronic fatigue, but is usually also accompanied by chronic muscle pain and insomnia. Life CFS, the causes of fibromyalgia are unknown and therefore traditional treatments are largely unavailable; however, there are some indications that aromatherapy may provide relief from the symptoms of both of these illnesses in many sufferers.

Tea tree oil (*Melaleuca alternifolia*) is an excellent choice as the primary treatment for both CFS and fibromyalgia. This special essential oil contains a wealth of potent remedial properties, including antiviral, antimicrobial and antifungal qualities. It also acts as a powerful immuno-stimulant, giving the body's natural disease and virus fighting system a good boost. Anecdotal evidence suggests that tea tree oil can yield positive results for the treatment of symptoms associated with both of these illnesses, and has even been shown to have a long term beneficial effect in some patients following ongoing use. Eucalyptus oil, meanwhile, can act as an effective stimulant in those experiencing bouts of fatigue. Peppermint, basil and rosemary can all also act as mental stimulants in the right quantities, which can lead to a patient feeling uplifted following treatment. These oils also have the effect of providing pain relief for those experiencing the muscular aches and pains associated with fibromyalgia. Finally, lavender once again can prove useful in this context due to its soothing effect and ability to relax mental fatigue. Not only can this be helpful in patients suffering with fatigue-based symptoms, but may also prove a beneficial treatment for those suffering with insomnia.

When creating a blend to apply during massage treatment for CFS or fibromyalgia, some experimentation can be in order using combinations of the abovementioned oils. Different patients may respond more favorably to certain essential oils, which may be due to the fact that these illnesses are thought to be caused by a number of different factors rather than one singular underlying pathology. Using a carrier oil high in essential fatty acids (EFAs) can also be a good course of treatment for CFS and fibromyalgia sufferers. The delivery of massage therapy using a blend containing a carrier oil rich in EFAs can be a wise course of action in such cases, as these important nutrients are vital for regulating proper brain and hormonal function. A great example of one such carrier is cranberry seed oil, which contains a good balance of omega-3, omega-6 and omega-9 fatty acids. Coconut oil can also be a good option thanks to its high levels of vitamins and minerals. Though the following may need to be tweaked for optimal results depending on the recipient, a good basic treatment for suffers of CFS or fibromyalgia involves: 4 drops of tea tree oil; 3 drops of eucalyptus oil; 3 drops of peppermint oil; 5mL of cranberry oil, and; 5mL of grapeseed oil. Combine all ingredients in a dark glass jar and shake well to emulsify. This blend can be applied via a chosen massage treatment and may be stored for up to 12 months.

The massage techniques used in delivering treatment for the above illnesses should follow a pattern likely to induce calming and relaxation. As such, a good potential massage treatment should involve light and repetitive techniques, such as effleurage and gentle tapotement. Lymphatic massage can also be a good option in this context, due to the strong correlation between a well-functioning lymphatic system and good health. This type of therapy involves stimulating the lymphatic system which is responsible for proper immune system function. The lymphatic system circulates a plasma-like substance throughout the body (known as *lymph*) which helps to clear waste products, cell debris, bacteria and protein from tissue throughout the body. An underperforming lymphatic system can precipitate chronic illness, and a series of good lymphatic massages can be just the thing to kick start the immune system. Though it is recommended that one undertakes specialized in person training to learn the art of lymphatic massage, the following is a rough outline of basic lymphatic massage, and may be performed by amateur practitioners of therapeutic massage without notable adverse effect. Lymphatic massage is typically gentle and slow in nature, as its primary goal is to gently and repetitively stimulate the lymphatic system, rather than manipulate muscle tissue. The locational focus of lymphatic massage is typically on the upper body, arms, neck and face, and the strokes of this type of massage move in the direction of the flow of the lymphatic system. The particulars of lymphatic massage are a little too complicated to explain here (as mentioned above, if you have an interest in performing this type of massage it is perhaps best to receive thorough guidance from a trained practitioner); however, an online search for '*Simple Lymphatic Drainage*' will yield many useful diagrams, videos and schematics that can guide the amateur masseuse in performing a rudimentary form of lymphatic massage.

It goes without saying that care should be taken in administering any treatment to severely ill patients, as massage therapy may indeed worsen some advanced illnesses. Patients who are experiencing chronic illness should consult their physician to determine whether aromatherapy treatments are safe and suitable for them on a case by case basis.

Chapter 7 – Meditation

One of the great complements between massage and aromatherapy is the ability of both treatments to deliver intense feelings of relaxation for the recipient. The reasons for this occurrence are manifold. The rhythmic, repetitive motion of massage has many parallels with the practice of mindfulness-based meditation. Not only does the action of massage release chemicals that can help calm our minds and nervous systems, but it can also be rather easy to begin to mentally drift into wonderful nothingness during a massage, relaxing the mind and the body by intensely (yet often subconsciously) focusing on the serenity of the moment. This explains the natural link between ancient eastern religions and massage, wherein the practice of meditation is also usually held in high regard. Many essential oils used in the practice of aromatherapy, meanwhile, can have a similarly potent effect in inducing feelings of relaxation in a subject.

Some suitable essential oils for use during a treatment focused on meditation include those that induce focus, alertness and calm in a patient. These include frankincense, cedarwood, sandalwood and rosemary. Frankincense is renowned for its ability to induce mental alertness and focus, and has been shown to improve concentration after repeated use in some patients. Sandalwood is also a wonderful aid for improving concentration, while cedarwood and rosemary are beneficial when it comes to inducing relaxation. When creating an aromatherapy blend to be used during meditation, this balance between concentration and relaxation is important when it comes to inducing the delicate mental state required for successful meditation to occur.

When complemented with some mindfulness techniques, this treatment can produce amazing results in those experiencing high levels of stress. This can include encouraging a subject to focus on the sensation of the massage therapy and nothing else (which will become easier after continued sessions). Clinical studies suggest that there is a definite link between practicing mindfulness and lowering stress levels. One such study indicated that those who took part in a 12 week mindfulness course showed significant changes in the size of the amygdala (the brain's fear and emotion center), as indicated by MRI scans taken before and after the 12 week period. In theory, a smaller amygdala will result in a less easily stimulated stress response. This highlights the positive effect that meditative practice can have on our overall wellbeing, and highlight the potential advantage of meditative massage.

When it comes to marrying massage, aromatherapy and mindfulness therapy, there is perhaps no better treatment available than the raindrop technique. Pioneered by Dr Gary Young during the 1980s, this specially constructed massage technique combines three distinct treatments into one holistic therapy: aromatherapy, the *Vita Flex* technique, and feather stroking. In summary, the raindrop technique involves applying essential oils to the neck, spine and feet. This treatment gets its name from the method in which the oils are applied; typically, they are 'dripped' onto the target areas from a height of about 6 inches, simulating the feeling of raindrops. The *Vita Flex* technique is based in ancient Tibetan healing practices, and involves the use of pressure applied to specific areas of the body. This is intended to stimulate an electrical impulse response at key points in the body, and make a patient more physiologically receptive to an aromatherapy treatment. The feather stroking component of this treatment is influenced by the ritual practices of the Lakota (Native American tribe) people, who used long strokes from a feather that was intended to act as a replication of the energy transmitted to a person during their exposure to the Northern Lights. These three distinct, yet complementary elements all have the effect of engaging a subject's body, mind and spirit, which makes it the perfect massage therapy for combining aromatherapy and meditation. For a visual instruction on how to perform this advanced form of massage, you should consult a video hosting website such as YouTube and carry out a search for the term *'raindrop technique massage'*.

Chapter 8 – Improving Circulation

There is little need to delve into statistical analyses or cite clinical research in order to understand that illnesses related to circulation problems affect vast swathes of the global population. Strokes, heart attacks and diabetes are just a few conditions that can be traced to circulation-related issues and affect millions of people each year. Poor circulation has a number of causes, and can result in a number of different symptoms, which may include numbness, coldness and tingling in the extremities; blue tinged lips and nail beds; tiredness and a lack of energy; headaches and dizziness; shortness of breath, and; irregularities in blood vessels (e.g. varicose veins). There is, however, somewhat of a disconnect when it comes to appreciating just how serious poor circulation problems can be in terms of overall health. Often, the symptoms of poor circulation are a cry for help from our bodies, a signal that there is a serious problem somewhere within that is making areas that the body sees as less valuable slow down and become damaged. Over time, problems with circulation can become severe, resulting in complete loss of feeling in the affected area which can lead to wounds and infections occurring, limb death, and in the most severe scenarios, a fatal episode such as a massive stroke or heart attack. In severe cases of paralysis in the extremities, nerve damage caused by poor circulation can be irreparable. Fortunately, however, there are a number of essential oils which exhibit special circulation boosting properties and help to rectify problems associated with restricted blood flow. Massage therapy, meanwhile, is particularly effective for encouraging regular blood flow throughout the treated area.

Essential oils that help to promote normal circulation include chamomile, ginger, geranium and cypress. Already discussed in some detail in previous chapters, chamomile oil is a good choice for aromatherapy treatments aimed at improving circulation. This is perhaps due to the strong anti-inflammatory properties of the oil, which can have an effect in reducing swelling in blood vessels. Ginger oil is particularly effective when it comes to stimulating blood flow, as it contains a range of amino acids and minerals that help to thin the blood, and belongs to the family of so-called 'hot oils' which all have good circulation boosting properties (such as peppermint, clove or cinnamon, for example). The underutilized hazelnut oil is a great boon for improving circulation as part of an aromatherapy blend as it is easily absorbed and has powerful astringent properties (which causes constriction of bodily tissues, more easily drawing oils into the bloodstream). As such, a good blend to be used in a circulation enhancing massage may include: 3 drops of chamomile oil; 2 drops of ginger oil; 3 drops of geranium oil; 2 drops of cypress oil; 10mL of hazelnut oil. This blend should be prepared by collecting ingredients in a dark glass jar and shaking well to combine.

As all forms of massage can provide a decent boost to blood flow, any massage is a good massage when it one is aiming to improve circulation. However, lymphatic massage (discussed earlier in Chapter 7) can be particularly effective in improving general circulation. As the lymphatic system comprises a key part of the circulatory system, its proper flow and function is important for the regulation of the circulatory system as a whole. Please refer to the abovementioned chapter for further advice on how to perform lymphatic massage. In general, any firm massage is useful when attempting to stimulate blood flow throughout the body. In terms of the Swedish massage methods, tapotement is particularly effective for inducing improved circulation and may be applied throughout the body of the patient. Please note, however, that massage treatment should generally be avoided in patients who have a history of thrombosis, as vigorous massage therapy may lead to the disruption of blood clots which may lead to stroke.

Chapter 9 – Headaches

Although many people are probably more inclined to reach for a packet of painkillers than to think of massage when it comes to alleviating the pain of a headache, this alternative treatment can actually be highly effective in terms of providing relief from pressure headaches and migraines. Many people tend to associate headaches with pain signals emanating from the brain itself; however, the brain actually lacks the necessary pain receptors to signal pain in that organ. 'Brain pain', therefore, doesn't really exist, and is certainly not what we are feeling when a headache occurs. Instead, headaches are typically the result of pain signals being sent by structures surrounding the brain, such as the blood vessels, nerves, subcutaneous tissues and mucous membranes found in and around the cranium. Massage and aromatherapy can be used to effectively address many of the complaints associated with these pain sensitive areas, and can often improve or eliminate headaches entirely.

The holy trinity of essential oils when it comes to the treatment of headaches consists of lavender, peppermint and basil oils. These three oils work in harmony to induce calming and general relaxation, improve circulation and induce muscle relaxation. The calming properties of lavender have been discussed earlier and are important for targeting headaches that may be caused by high levels of stress. Peppermint oil is great for regulating blood flow throughout the treated area, thanks to its complementary vasoconstricting and vasodialiting properties. Basil oil, meanwhile, acts as an effective muscle relaxant and can help to relieve headaches that are brought on by muscle tension. For a comprehensive headache treatment, these oils should be combined with a nourishing blend, such as avocado oil, which can have the bonus effect of providing important nutrients for the skin.

An excellent massage treatment for the alleviation of headaches is an advanced massage therapy that is known as *'Indian head massage'*. This type of massage has been born from centuries of tradition and is based on traditional ancient Ayurvedic healing techniques. In particular, this massage involves the massage of the upper back, neck, arms, head and face, and is effective for both increasing circulation and reducing tension in the targeted area, both of which can be a source of headaches. During this treatment, the recipient is normally seated upright and may remain fully clothed. Specific strokes and techniques during and Indian head massage include muscle compression, deep kneading, and the manipulation of pressure points in the different focal areas. It is generally recommended to move through the massage in sections, starting with the back, shoulders and arms, then progressing to the neck, scalp and the face. While this treatment can vary in its level of technicality, however, a few of the abovementioned basic massage techniques (such as effleurage, petrissage and tapotement) can be utilized in a basic form of Indian head massage. Furthermore, although this specific kind of massage treatment is best delivered after thorough training and instruction, there are a couple key points to keep in mind if trying to deliver this kind of therapy at home. First, it is important to be gentle (but firm) when practicing this type of massage as it involves areas that are particularly sensitive (especially the face and neck). For that reason it is also important to make sure that the patient notifies the masseur at the first sign of any discomfort during the treatment. Additionally, it is advisable to avoid applying anything more than light pressure to the face or neck unless the masseur has received thorough training in the art of pressure point massage.

Conclusion

As the above has shown, there is almost limitless potential when it comes to the possible therapeutic application of essential oils via massage. Though this book has highlighted just a few of the potential applications of this pairing, there are countless possibilities when it comes to remedying health complaints using these methods. One of the beauties of this treatment combination is the fact that the healing properties of the essential oils complement the therapeutic power of massage (and vice versa) remarkably well, leading to some highly effective remedies for a number of health-related conditions.

For those interested in honing their massage skills further, it is highly recommended to engage with additional resources that can provide further insight and instruction for developing technique and perfecting massage execution. A good place to start is with online resources. There are a number of useful instructional videos that can be found online simply by searching for suitable terms, such as 'aromatherapy massage pain relief', for example. As certain types of massage can be highly technical, it is almost always a good idea to try and see the type of massage you plan to carry out in practice before performing it on your own.

Another good idea when it comes to developing your aromatherapy massage technique further is to sign up for a course of personal instruction. There are many holistic therapy schools that offer special courses on the subject and, in the author's opinion, are essential for those wishing to take their practice of this discipline to the next level. It can even be a good idea for those interested in aromatherapy massage to attend a few sessions of therapy with a trained practitioner and simply observe their practice and techniques. As with the wider world of aromatherapy, there is much to learn when it comes to aromatherapy, and, as with many such arts, one stands to learn the most from those who are already masters in the field.

While this guide has not been an exhaustive introduction into the world of aromatherapy massage, with the information contained herein I hope to have given you enough information to confidently begin exploring this wonderful marriage. As with our previous book (an introduction to essential oils and aromatherapy) this guide should be viewed as a building block for a newcomer's aromatherapy education, and will hopefully encourage readers to explore a little on their own. Be sure to keep an eye out for future books in this series which will help you to build your foundational knowledge of aromatherapy to even greater heights.

2 FREE eBooks for you!

Guys, thanks so much for reading my book. I truly hope it served as a great introduction to the essential oils and aromatherapy. As a token of appreciation I have prepared two free ebooks for you. Here is a bit of information about them!

The 10 Most Important Essential Oils

In this book we delve deep into the uses and applications of the ten essential oils that I consider to be the most 'essential'. It is the natural progression from this beginner's guide that you have just read. For each oil I explain the key health benefits, teach you the therapeutic applications and provide specific safety precaution. I include one of my most useful remedies for each of the oils as well. So you will receive a deep knowledge of ten essential oils and ten brilliant remedies for free! It is a 10k word eBook, the same length as this one!

When you receive this ebook you will also receive a couple of emails from me a week containing even more information about the essential oils! I will endeavour to give you at least 5 recipes or remedies per week and also provide you with some great information on the lesser known essential oils.

Simply type this link into a web browser: http://bit.ly/1EuHgyn

The Ultimate Guide To Vitamins

This is another wonderful 10k word ebook that has been made available to you through my publisher, Valerian Press. As a health conscious person you should be well aware of the uses and health benefits of each of the vitamins that should make up our diet. This book gives you an easy to understand, scientific explanation of the vitamin followed by the recommended daily dosage. It then highlights all the important health benefits of each vitamin. A list of the best sources of each vitamin is provided and you are also given some actionable next steps for each vitamin to make sure you are utilizing the information!

As well as receiving the free ebooks you will also be sent a weekly stream of free ebooks, again from my publishing company Valerian Press. You can expect to receive at least a new, free ebook each and every week. Sometimes you might receive a massive 10 free books in a week!

Simply type this link into a web browser: http://bit.ly/1EuHgyn

Preview of "Essential Oils For Beginners"

I have included an example chapter of my first book here to give you a taste of the content. I really would recommend reading this book to gain a well-rounded understanding of the essential oils! Find it here:

http://www.amazon.com/dp/B00T12QLW4

Alternatively you can simply search for Amy Joyson in the Kindle Store and it will pop right up!

"What are essential oils?

Simply put, essential oils are the concentrated essences (hence, the use of the term 'essential') of aromatic compounds. In Ancient China, these plant and flower essences were believed to constitute the 'soul' of the organism. These are often clear liquids and, contrary to the 'oil' in their name, often have a consistency more like that of water than of typical oils. From herbs, to flowers, to fruits, essential oils can be derived from many different organic sources. Around 400-500 essential oils are produced commercially, although there are many more types available. Essential oils are typically very complex, with single varieties often containing hundreds of individual aromatic compounds. As essential oils are derived from natural sources, they contain no harmful or synthetic chemicals which can have unknown detrimental effects on the body.

Essential oils are a key ingredient in many of today's consumer products, particularly in foodstuffs and cosmetics. They are also the subject around which the practice of aromatherapy is based. Essential oils hold great appeal to the individual due to their accessibility and usefulness. Not only can they be applied therapeutically, but also in foods, for household cleaning solutions, or simply for their distinctive aromatic properties. There are few tinctures which have such numerous practical applications, and are locked within the natural world that surrounds us, ready to be released.

How are essential oils obtained?

The process of extracting essential oils varies, largely depending upon the source material and available technologies. The oldest and perhaps simplest method of extracting essential oils is a process known as *enfleurage*. A relatively simple method, this involves crushing the product from which the oils are to be derived, and mixing the resulting powder or paste with a lipid (such as olive or vegetable oil). The oils from the source product permeate the lipids, and the essential oil infused mixture is then processed to be separated from the product residue. Though yielding a rather crude final result, this was a common method due to the lack of knowledge and expertise surrounding more complex extractions. The process for exploiting essential oils became more sophisticated over time. Archaeological evidence from the Middle East, such as pottery stills containing the residue of aromatic compounds, indicates that advanced extraction techniques were already being practiced in ancient times. Today, more sophisticated extraction methods mean that we can obtain highly pure and refined essential oils. The most pure essential oils are obtained through a process of steam distillation, whereby a solution is made from the source product, which is then heated, evaporating the essential oils. These are later collected through condensation after being cooled further along the system. The purity of essential oils is especially important when it comes to their therapeutic administration.

Another technique used for obtaining essential oils is the use of *solvents*. The use of chemical solvents is generally unfavorable amongst professional aromatherapists as it is the least natural way of extracting essential oils. The idea behind the method is that all the solvents used in the extraction are removed but occasionally light chemical traces will be left in the product. In this method the plant from which the essential oil is to be sourced is dissolved in a chemical solvent. The most common solvents used are; methylene chloride, hexane and benzene. These solvents have a lower boiling point than the essential oils and so are evaporated off, leaving behind the pure essential oil.

One of the most popular methods of obtaining essential oils is *steam distillation*. It is a simple procedure in which freshly harvested plants are suspended above a vat of boiling water. The steam that emerges from the water extracts the oil from the plant. The rising steam is captured and pushed through a tube before being cooled. As the steam condenses back into water, the essential oil (which doesn't mix with water) separates away.

Obtaining 'therapeutic grade' essential oils

In order to enjoy the therapeutic benefit of essential oils, it is vital that a product that is both high in purity and quality is used. However, essential oils that meet these requirements can be very expensive, due to the fact that a very high amount of organic matter is required to produce each milliliter of oil. In addition to this, it is much cheaper to extract the oils when sub-standard techniques are used. Typically, the extraction technique that results in the best quality oils requires both expensive distillation equipment and the expertise of a professional trained in its operation to perform the extraction. Sadly, the market for essential oils is severely lacking in regulation. Although, on the one hand this means that essential oils are readily obtainable, on the other, it makes certification of the quality of the product for sale difficult to verify for the individual. Therefore, as consumers of these important commodities, there are certain things we should look for, especially when shopping online for essential oils for therapeutic use:

- Is the information relating to the product thoroughly and adequately provided? E.g. Is the Latin name of the plant genus provided? Is the source of origin of the extract given?

- Does the product information state that the oils are 100% pure? Is there a suggestion that oils have been adulterated with other substances?

- When you receive the product, is it adequately and correctly labelled? Does the product smell as you would expect it to smell?

- Is the product significantly cheaper than normal market prices? If so, it is likely that the quality or purity of the product is compromised. (If it seems too good to be true, it usually is)

- Does the vendor seem legitimate? Do they appear to be knowledgeable about the product they are selling? Does the vendor seem trustworthy?

- Is the vendor you are purchasing the product from well-reviewed? If possible, try to find review of the company by third parties rather than relying on those that appear on their own website.

Although it can be difficult to guarantee that we are buying a legitimate product, particularly when shopping online, this can be true of any item – not just essential oils. It is important to carry out these basic precautions to protect ourselves as consumers, and to ensure that we are using a product of the highest quality. Remember; if you have reasons to suspect that the quality of an essential oil you have purchased is compromised *do not administer it therapeutically!*

How much should I be paying for essential oils?

As alluded to above, the comparative price of an essential oil is almost always reflective of its quality. However, there is no 'set price' for essential oils as such. All differ based on the expensiveness of the source material from which they are derived, and the volume of material required to produce one milliliter of essential oil. For example, take the case of essence of lemon. A large number of lemons are indeed required to produce one standard bottle of essence of lemon; however, because lemons are relatively inexpensive, it is normally one of the cheaper essential oils. A suggestion would be to compare the price of the oil you are looking to purchase to other reputable sites on the internet to make sure the price is in line.

How are essential oils administered?

Essential oils can be administered in a number of different ways. One of the most basic and effective methods (depending on the symptom being treated) is through topical application. This is not only true for treating topical conditions (e.g. such as skin irritation or bruising) but is also often a way to treat internal complaints (e.g. such as headaches or nausea). This method is connected to perhaps one of the most traditional ways to deliver therapeutic treatment in conjunction with massage therapy. When applied to the skin, essential oils are absorbed relatively quickly, as they are made up of very small molecules that are easily drawn into the dermis. This means that they are able to enter the bloodstream and take effect very quickly, compared to other therapeutic treatments.

A second way to administer essential oils is via either direct or indirect inhalation. In the case of the former, a personal inhaler is loaded with the oil(s) and their vapor is inhaled through the nose or mouth. For the latter, a vaporizer is typically employed, where the vapor of the oil(s) is diffused throughout a room. These methods are often best when treating an issue related to respiratory function, colds or flus, or sinus complaints. The final and perhaps least common method of administering essential oils is via ingestion. Though this technique can be suitable to obtain specific therapeutic results, it can be less safe than the above methods, particularly when not practiced or prescribed by a trained professional. Certain essential oils can damage the liver or kidneys when taken internally, or can interact with certain medications. Additionally, contraindications can occur when essential oils are processed through the digestive system. Always seek the advice of a trained professional if planning to administer essential oils via this method.

How do essential oils work?

From the three main ways that essential oils enter the body (dermally, or through inhalation or ingestion), the active ingredients interact with the body's systems in different ways. When taken through the skin, or via ingestion, the compounds from essential oils enter the blood stream acting much like a regular drug. They then circulate throughout the body and can have a localized effect on symptoms. Also when ingested, the ingredients from the oils are processed through the digestive system before being circulated through blood to the rest of the body.

When inhaled through the nose or mouth, essential oils interact with a number of different systems in the body. The olfactory system is responsible for controlling and effecting the sense of smell. As essential oils are highly aromatic, their interaction with the olfactory system can be an important part of their therapeutic application. Inhaled molecules also interact directly with the respiratory system, which can be a useful method of delivery when treating complaints associated with the respiratory tract and the lungs.

Finally, inhaled oils are believed to achieve some of their therapeutic outcomes by interacting with various receptors in the brain which constitute the limbic system. This system is thought to be responsible for a range of physiological responses, including heart rate, blood pressure, memory, breathing, and stress and hormone levels. This helps to explain why essential oils can have a profound array of effects on both human physiology and emotional well-being.

Why aren't essential oils backed as 'therapeutic drugs' by federal regulators?

One of the main issues surrounding universal acceptance of the 'therapeutic drug' status of essential oils relates to the dearth of clinical research evidence associated with them. However, this is not due to a lack of a link between essential oils and quantifiable therapeutic effect, but is primarily related to the fact that the number of clinical studies actually conducted in the area of essential oils has been limited. Many advocates of the therapeutic properties of essential oils claim that this is a result of two key factors. The first is due to the fact that drug companies have limited interest in sponsoring clinical trials in this area, due to a limited potential for profit. There is little to no money to be made from essential oils within the pharmaceutical industry, as they are natural products derived from natural sources, and therefore, are not patentable. Patents on drug design and manufacture are the number one source of revenue in the pharmaceutical industry.

Relatedly, the process for having drugs tested and certified by federal drug regulators is typically prohibitively expensive and depends upon the backing of the multibillion dollar pharmaceutical industry in some form. Thus, because backing by federal drug regulators *and* the pharmaceutical industry (who, because of the above may see the widespread therapeutic use of essential oils as contrary to their financial interests) are requisite for mainstream acceptance of therapeutic treatments, essential oils face a legitimacy problem. However, thanks to the limited clinical studies which *have* been conducted into essential oils thus far, we know that many of these products do in fact have clear antibacterial, antiviral and antifungal properties. This means that they can have a quantifiable effect on treating certain illnesses and conditions. Additionally, studies conducted on laboratory animals have shown that exposure to certain aromas under stressful conditions can improve behavioral and immune response. Finally, the amount of anecdotal evidence surrounding the positive therapeutic effects of essential oils is enormous. While not certifiable (as in the case of clinical evidence), this widespread popular backing nonetheless suggests that a significant multitude of people have used essential oils with great therapeutic results."

The book can be found here:
http://www.amazon.com/dp/B00T12QLW4